ONE VICTOR'S
STORY

*Moving From Victim To Victory When
Facing A Devastating Diagnosis*

VINCENT STEPHENS, JR.

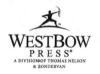

WESTBOW
P R E S S®
A DIVISION OF THOMAS NELSON
& ZONDERVAN

This book is a work of non-fiction. Unless otherwise noted, the author and the publisher make no explicit guarantees as to the accuracy of the information contained in this book and in some cases, names of people and places have been altered to protect their privacy.

WestBow Press books may be ordered through booksellers or by contacting:

WestBow Press
A Division of Thomas Nelson & Zondervan
1663 Liberty Drive
Bloomington, IN 47403
www.westbowpress.com
1 (866) 928-1240

ISBN: 978-1-5127-9662-9 (sc)
ISBN: 978-1-5127-9663-6 (hc)
ISBN: 978-1-5127-9664-3 (e)

Library of Congress Control Number: 2017911469

Print information available on the last page.

WestBow Press rev. date: 08/07/2017

CONTENTS

INTRODUCTION

For the past 37 years, I have answered letters and phone calls regarding my health condition. I have multiple sclerosis. I was one of the unfortunate who suffered from most every problem MS could cause. I was one of the unfortunate who did everything the doctor suggested. I was also one of the fortunate who discovered a way to control my condition.

This book is written for those with MS and other degenerative conditions who don't understand that I haven't the time or money to personally respond to their questions. This book is written for those who treated me medically. This book is written for those who had to live with me. This book is written not out of vanity, but out of need. Most information presently available about MS seems to be written by professionals who study the condition. I felt it was time for a book written by someone living with it.

When I was diagnosed as having MS, I was given the news that I would become progressively worse. I had no idea of the thousands of people suffering from MS living relatively normal lives. I felt that life was over for me. I suffered depression, anger, frustration, and confusion. My health did just as the doctors suggested it would. I got worse day by day. I was not able to find any success stories of those who beat the problem.

That's why this book is written. It is a book of hope for all those who suffer with MS and other degenerative conditions. I am not writing this book as a prescription to anyone suffering from MS. I am not saying this is the way to cure MS. *I am not cured.* I am not saying this will work for everyone. I am simply outlining what happened to me and how I dealt with it. Some may read this and feel it is simply a "placebo effect". Quite possibly it is. But it worked!

I am not medically trained. I have no degree that gives me the right to prescribe. But as a victim of MS, I feel I am entitled to my own opinion and the right to express it.

This book is written with the sincere hope of good health for everyone. Read it with the dream and the hope that something in it will help you.

CHAPTER

1

Until my senior year of high school, I had no complaints. I was enjoying life to its fullest. My parents were financially secure and able to provide all I could want. I suppose you could say I was even a bit spoiled. I had a 1965 Mustang with a fast engine in it I had built. I used the engine in that car to win at area race tracks. I had a steady girlfriend. I played bass in the local symphony and even played in a rock-and-roll band. It was the bass playing that gave me my first clue that things weren't right.

One night in the spring of 1970, the band was playing a concert promoting our second record. I was not able to play my part with the same speed and precision I used when we recorded the song. I blamed it on the fact that I had been drinking all day. Actually, it seemed I drank a lot while I was in the band. So I stopped drinking for a while but the tremors in my hands persisted and my dexterity seemed off as I played. My parents also noticed the problem when they watched me eating or drinking and made an appointment for me with our family doctor.

When I got to his office, I told him about my problems playing my bass guitar and demonstrated how my hands quivered. He asked if I was taking drugs. I told him honestly that I had never done any chemical or hallucinatory drugs. We discussed the hours I spent with the band at night and how early I got up in the morning to be at school. He said he could see no physical problem. It appeared I was trying to do too much and needed to slow down. Having the assurance from one in the medical profession there was no major problem, I continued my lifestyle. After all, it's useless to tell a teenager to slow down and take it easy.

Being 17, I also had the usual amount of romance in my life. I had a steady girlfriend. I also dated other girls when she and I were fighting or separated by miles due to vacation or the music. My dating others always upset her, and one day she confronted me wanting to know why I ran around on her so much. I replied it was for the memories, "Someday I might be crippled, in a wheelchair and women won't have anything to do with me. I can think back to when I played in the band and had them all over me."

It was a very arrogant response. I spent much time in later years wondering if my health problems were payment for my casual attitude toward everything and everyone. I was young and concerned about nothing but my own happiness.

After graduation from high school, I went to Dallas for the summer. My father was opening another restaurant. I had visions of stepping into his business with him. A friend of mine lived in a lake shore home and we spent much time that summer water skiing. Each time I finished skiing, the ankle that supported my weight would go crazy with a violent tremor. I thought I was simply out of shape.

Later that summer, my father noticed my arm shaking as I tried to drink a glass of orange juice. He did not accept my assurance that it did it all the time and insisted I see his doctor. This doctor decided I was taking life too seriously and worried too much. He gave me a powerful tranquilizer. That night when my father came home, he saw me standing there glassy eyed and smiling and said "What did he give you? You look doped up!"

I showed him the bottle of prescription tranquilizers. He promptly threw them away declaring there was nothing wrong with me.

With fall approaching, it became college time. I decided I would return to my home in Kansas and go to the local junior college the first year. I wasn't ready to leave my friends, music and race track. I enrolled in school working toward a business degree.

In early November of 1970, as I was running laps in gym class, my legs became numb. I stopped and as the circulation returned, the numbness left. I jogged into the showers and went on to my next class. I was not scared now, I was terrified. As I thought back on the numbness, the weak ankle, and the shaking hands, I knew something was definitely wrong. One of my courses was a basic health class which I viewed as an easy credit. That afternoon in class, we were assigned a chapter about an illness I had never heard of, multiple sclerosis. The text book described the illness as a nervous disorder characterized by numbness in the arms and legs, coordination problems, and tremors. It gave no cause or cure but I didn't even notice that. I knew this had to be my problem, and I could do nothing but smile thinking that now I knew what was wrong with me.

That afternoon, I went back to my doctor without an appointment. When he walked into the reception area, I approached him and asked if he thought I might have multiple sclerosis. He stopped with a sick look on his face and said, "My God, I never thought of that. Go into my examination room and I will be with you in a minute." All of a sudden, for some reason, I didn't feel so good about all of this. The doctor returned and checked my reflexes. They were very hypersensitive. He chatted with me about how I learned of multiple sclerosis. He said "it looks possible but I'm not qualified to make that diagnosis." He would talk to my parents and get me scheduled to see a specialist in Wichita who was qualified in this area.

That night I went to see my girlfriend. I told her quite casually I thought I had MS. She buried her head in her hands and then ran from the room crying. I asked her mother what was wrong and learned that her grandmother had died from MS the previous year. I didn't remember reading this thing was fatal! I tried to calm her down and convince her I wasn't going to die. Now all I had to do was convince myself.

In less than a week. I was checked into a Wichita hospital for ten days of testing. The first test was a spinal tap. They explained it was being done to determine the percentage of gamma globulin in my spinal fluid. I was told that normal content was around 12%. If mine tested at 15 to 30% I had MS.

My test results showed 6%. The doctor felt that with the content this low it must be a brain tumor. It's strange, but that sounded good to me. You see, they could remove brain tumors and then that would be that!

If I sound cocky and sure of a solution, I wasn't. When my girlfriend came with her mother to visit me in the hospital I was very rude to them. I didn't want sympathy and didn't want to hurt one so close to me with my problems. My dad drove up from Oklahoma to see me. He had no other children and wasn't ready for what was happening. When he met my doctor and was told I had some sort of brain disorder. I thought he was going to punch the doctor in the nose!

Looking for a tumor, they gave me a pneumoencephalogram, a surgical type of brain scan. This was in 1970, well before the painless, sophisticated brain scans of today were developed. To do this test, they removed my spinal fluid in a complete spinal tap. Then they pumped air up through my spinal column into my brain cavities. As the air surrounded my brain, they took x-rays that were supposed to show any blockage from a tumor. Next they pulled the air out and replaced the spinal fluid. Until my body regenerated the spinal fluid missing in the crevices around my brain, I had an excruciating headache that worsened when I sat up or stood.

The next night was the ninth day in the hospital, and my parents were there to learn the results. When the doctor came in, my mother asked him what he had learned from the tests? He started hedging around and asked if they wanted him to discuss it in front of me. My step-father said I was a big boy and could take it. The conversation that followed quickly knocked away my hopes for a simple cure. My mother and I could only listen in disbelief as the doctor and my step-father talked.

"I've already told you I don't think its MS, and the brain scan didn't show me the location of a tumor."

"What does that mean?"

"That means it's inoperable."

"Is it fatal?"

"I would say the way he's progressing, he has between ten minutes and two years to live."

"Do you mean he's dying?"

The doctor nodded his head.

"Can we do anything?"

"Yes, he can take ACTH, which is a form of cortisone, that I treat my MS patients with and it could slow the tumor's growth."

"Is the tumor malignant?"

"No, it's a benign, slow growing tumor."

Even now, as I look back to that evening, I have no memory of anything between that conversation and the trip home the next day. The hour drive was anything but happy. Everyone seemed trapped in their own silent thoughts.

I was rather numb from the news I was dying. I had a terrible headache from the brain scan, and I had developed an attitude of "what next?" and "who cares?" At least I had a good idea of what my future was going to be, soon ended!

For the next week, I spent most of my time lying around listening to very loud rock and roll through stereo headphones.

Somehow, I didn't feel like I was dying. In fact, I'd never felt so alive.

My parents, who never gave up, had a friend whose son was an intern at Mayo Clinic in Rochester, Minnesota. This was definitely a case of who you know. We had an open appointment for whenever we could get there. My mother and I flew to Rochester on November 18th, 1970. I made sure we had the pneumoencephalogram with us and made it clear to my mother I would not let them do that test to me again.

In two days Mayo Clinic made a diagnosis. The head of the Neurological Department said there wasn't any brain tumor and although it didn't appear to be MS, that was all it could be.

Finally we had a diagnosis, not just a guess. And any way you looked at it, Mayo Clinic said Vince Stephens had MS and wasn't going to die. At least not from a brain tumor. My problems were far from over, but now I had plenty of time to figure them out and try to solve them. I think Mom and I laughed most of the way home on the airplane about silly stuff that wasn't even funny. It was much different than the return from Wichita.

2

The next four years were quite an experience. The fact I had this terrible health problem created many changes in my life. I became very uncertain about education and finally ended school entirely. I became a part of the working world. There didn't seem to be much sense in a college degree when the doctors kept telling me I would just get worse. I ended my serious relationship with my girlfriend. What was the purpose in feeling I could offer her much in life? Better to let her go. I became quite casual in my relationships, allowing myself the pleasure of contact but not the responsibility of commitment. I changed jobs and found myself in the high pressure position of collections for a finance company. This seemed good to me. They moved me often so I didn't have to stay anywhere and form a serious relationship. It also kept me away from my family so they didn't see me every day and worry about me.

I could see new doctors all the time and take anything and everything they had to offer as help. And they did try to help. The problem was that there is no cure for MS, there is no treatment for MS. There are only doctors who want to help and

going to be laid off since the company was afraid of liability for any accident I might have at work. I didn't want to be fired, so I quit and went on disability insurance. I decided to enjoy retirement. It was 1974 and I was 21.

I don't remember the next year very well. I drank a lot, I fooled around a lot, and I went into the hospital for ACTH treatments several times. I tried any drug the doctor offered. In the fall of 1975 I moved in with a girl I was dating. Shortly after that my doctor began giving me the maximum dosage of Sodium Dantrolene, or Dantrium as it is more commonly known. But the tremors continued. In April of 1976 I began seeing double and quit driving. In May I did what I told myself I'd never do, after crawling for six months, I got a wheelchair. Ten days later I married the girl I was living with.

CHAPTER

3

If I am going to speak of marriage and love. I will have to say that my deepest emotions and thoughts of love were for my high school sweetheart. No one had equaled her. I had no business getting married. Between that and my MS my wife entered into a very painful relationship.

I guess that until now, I hadn't accepted MS for what it was and I certainly hadn't accepted it for what it could be. What was happening to me didn't make sense. Why was it happening? Sitting in the wheelchair I felt I could walk, but if I tried, I just couldn't do it. I hadn't wanted this wheelchair. I removed the foot rests from it so I would have to move my legs as I rolled around. My parents wanted to get me an electric wheelchair to make it easier, but I didn't want it to be easier. I wanted it to be over.

Why did I spill half the time when I took a drink? Why could I listen to music, know how to play it and not be able to even hold my guitar? What was God doing to me and why? I had coped with this for five and a half years and now I was 24 and *mad!* Why couldn't I lose my mind? Why did I have to remain so aware of what was happening to me? Up until now this had been like a joke, maybe a bad joke, but now there wasn't anything funny.

When things are going wrong and there is no one or nothing to blame, you blame whoever is closest. That happened to be my wife. She lived with the darkest side of me possible. I hope there is something special for her in the future. She deserves it.

That fall my dad heard of a doctor in Dallas who was experimenting with hormones to treat MS. I flew to Oklahoma City and drove to Dallas with my dad. The treatment given was injections of Depo-Provera which is a form of estrogen, a female sex hormone. I didn't think I needed female sex hormones, but I was desperate and ready to try anything. He gave me an injection of Depo-Provera and one of Depo-Testerone Extradiol. It worked fantastically. When I rolled into his office I couldn't even hold a pen because my tremors were so bad. Shortly after the injection I was signing my name. I even drove the car back to Oklahoma City that evening. It sure felt great to be rid of the tremors and double vision.

The doctor sent a prescription for the drugs along with me. Two days later I needed another injection. A day and a half later I needed another. Within two weeks the drugs had no effect except for three months of impotence. Years later I would read about the drugs this doctor gave me being used to chemically castrate rapists in our penal system.

My wife read everything she could find about MS. I kept going to the neurologist in Denver and taking anything he could offer. Friends and family smuggled drugs from overseas that were being used in other countries to treat MS. Nothing helped.

In the fall of 1976, my mother heard of a woman in Kansas City who had MS and used a treatment of vitamins to go from bedridden to healthy. She supposedly had regained the ability to drive a car and was doing great. I didn't know if this was fact or not but I know that people believe what they want to believe. I wanted to believe that this was it. And I hadn't heard of such recoveries with medical treatments. Anyway, by now I could only sit in the wheelchair and shake. I couldn't hold my head up. I lost my speech after I was given Clonopin. I had uncontrollable arching movements of my limbs. I couldn't feed myself. I couldn't do anything. My wife had to feed me, bathe me, brush my teeth, dress me, take me to the bathroom, the list was endless. Physically, I had no control at all.

We found a local distributor of the same brand of vitamins that this Kansas City woman had used for her recovery. But this really seemed different. I was told these weren't vitamins like you buy in a grocery store. They were called food supplements. These were whole food sources from organically grown produce. These could not hurt me anymore than overeating would hurt me. The distributor said there was no recommended dosage, but I should just take all I could. I chose to believe her.

I started taking 192 tablets a day. I had such bad tremors that my wife had to hold my head against her body and give me one tablet at a time. Depending on my tremors and how much I choked it took 20 to 40 minutes, six times a day. I was determined to give this the same chance I'd given chemical drugs the doctors had prescribed.

I was told it was a healthy sign when my body broke out in hives. According to the woman we got the supplements from, this meant my body was cleansing itself. I was even convinced to replace my daily enema with an herbal laxative. It worked just as well with less discomfort.

My neurologist in Denver told me he didn't think the vitamin program would help me, but he admitted it couldn't hurt. He ran blood tests and determined I was normal. What was normal? The government's RDA standards? What was normal? What some agency established as proper for anyone over 4 years old? I chose to ignore his findings of "normal". After all, maybe I wasn't doing better, but I felt better.

In December of 1977, I went to the hospital for my sixth treatment of ACTH. This was to be my last medical treatment. When the series was finished, I felt no better. My doctors had no other ideas for treatment. I decided to give the nutritional approach my full attention.

When I told the doctor my plans he tried to discourage me from pursuing it at all. He told me my medications should be tapered off from very slowly, by just stopping them it could kill me. I felt the drugs themselves were killing me. I went home and did a very foolish thing. I threw all my prescription drugs away. I wouldn't suggest my actions to anyone. I went through drug withdrawal. I ached, I sweated, I cried, I begged my wife to take my life. Then one day the pain left and I felt good again.

I still wasn't doing any better, but I wasn't doing any worse, and I wasn't taking the drugs. I didn't need them.

Having made the commitment to nutrition, I could only continue on my current program. I kept taking the supplements and we read all we could find on a nutritional approach to healing. The name of a doctor in West Germany kept turning up in articles about MS. My wife wrote him, asking how he was having success in treating MS, while doctors in America could do nothing. We read that patients checked into his clinic in my condition and walked out completely healthy. He sent us a reply that talked about his treatment being a nutritional one. His patients ate everything uncooked. He kept his patients away from foods cooked in oils or animal fats and served the foods raw to keep the highest nutritional value in them.

I decided that the supplements I was taking would substitute for the nutritional value lost in cooking. Anyway, his last statement in his letter had cautioned me against using his treatment in the United States. He said we used so many chemicals here to grow crops and raise livestock that a diet of our foods in a raw state might be "suicidal". I had never given any thought to how food was grown. I didn't realize that our livestock was being fed hormones and steroids to speed up their growth and limit fat. I hadn't given much thought to the danger of the pesticides and fertilizers used on our crops.

But his letter did make me decide to stay with my current program. I decided to try all those things that didn't involve doctors and chemical drugs. I became one of those "nutrition nuts".

My MS had made me unable to take the summer heat. I took a cold whirlpool treatment twice a day during the hot weather. I also tried a treatment called kinesiology that relaxed me as much as any tranquilizer, but I can't say it helped on a lasting basis.

I also tried chiropractors and acupuncture. One helpful chiropractor suggested leaving flour, sugar and red meat out of my diet. This was a major diet change but I did it. I couldn't eat anything I used to eat. I couldn't go to restaurants. The amazing thing was that after I had been on this program a while I was feeling fantastic. I just wasn't doing any better. I knew I was getting better, but I couldn't convince anyone of that fact.

In July of 1979 I was served divorce papers. Who could blame her? She had three years of marriage to someone who did nothing but scream at her in a garbled voice. I loved her but I wasn't over my high school romances. She went through three years of this. She had acted as a nurse and also tried to work full time. As my health had deteriorated, she had taken the full blame for it from me. I had been demanding, obstinate, argumentative and hard to live with. I don't think I would have lasted three years had the situation been reversed. I joined the ever growing group of MS people who found themselves divorced and alone.

My parents moved me back to their home in Kansas, but I didn't want to do to them what I had done to my wife. So I found a ground level apartment that was wheelchair accessible. I hired a woman to come in three times a day to feed me and a man to come in every evening to bathe me. I had my independence. I was not being a care problem for my family. I could continue my search for nutritional answers to MS.

I was sent an article about a man in England who had lost his sight and become paralyzed by MS. He had used a diet and supplement program to regain his health. I knew it had worked for others and I knew it would work for me. I was discovering the secret to the entire matter, attitude. Through all my reading I had learned that others had eliminated sugar, glutens and red meats. They were taking supplements, not chemical vitamins, but whole food sources. I was doing all of this as well. My family thought I was crazy, but I could feel it was working.

I kept my progress to myself. I held on to the foot board of my bed and did deep knee bends daily to keep my muscles active. In January of 1980 I decided the time had come to get out of the wheelchair. I put it in the closet and started stumbling around my apartment on a walker. My tremors were still bad. I had to have 40 pounds of weight strapped onto the walker so I could control it. As I got better the weights came off. Soon it was just me and the walker.

I had a neighbor who was in a wheelchair due to polio. One day she asked me if I wanted to go to a church singles dance with her group. This struck me as really ridiculous. She was in a wheelchair, I was on a walker, and we were going to a dance. Why not! She convinced me we could at least get out and meet some new people. I had always had a very active social life in my wheelchair. I hadn't been in the public eye for almost four years without being in that chair.

Hello world, here's Vince Stephens! After ten years of going downhill, I'm coming back!

CHAPTER

4

This dance was almost a rebirth. I was out in public and although I needed a walker, I was standing! And this dance had a special surprise for me, I met the a girl I would marry.

She was there with a friend, I was there with a friend, and neither of us would have been there otherwise. We talked and we danced and then we started arguing about diet and supplements. It all started with a discussion of my health. She didn't disagree with my method just the brand of supplements I used. My big argument was that my brand was working!

We argued for the next four months. But we also must have agreed about a few things, because after four months, we got married.

I suppose it wasn't really that easy. But from the start there was just something between us that wouldn't let either of us walk away. We both needed friendship and it became obvious we each had strengths the other one needed. She cooked me sugar free, flour free, and meat free goodies that she brought

about eating on time and taking my supplements on time. When I'm late with either, I get shaky and it makes me remember the bad years. That's always enough to make me take time for my health.

And that's what it's all about. It's about keeping a good attitude, treating your body right and sharing your accomplishments with someone who cares. It lives with me every day. That's the secret, I don't live with it. I make it live with me!

CHAPTER

5

MS is a depressing illness that follows no rules. The symptoms are many or few. You may have minor problems that never get worse, or you might have progressively worse problems that finally put you in a wheelchair. You might be symptom free one day and have several problems the next day.

Some symptoms of MS are loss of coordination, numbness, weakness, double vision, loss of vision, slurred speech, tremors, loss of bladder or bowel control, stiffness, loss of sensation, periods of mild to severe problems, and partial or complete remissions. When you give these problems to someone in today's society, you can usually add loss of job, spouse, normal life, and income to the list.

MS is hard for family to understand. It's even harder for the MS victim to understand. The loss of sensation doesn't seem too important unless you happen to be a male and want to have a normal sex life. Suddenly sensation is very important to performance. Slurred speech doesn't seem too bad unless you have a job dealing with the public. Loss of bladder control is no real problem if you like to stay home all the time to spare yourself embarrassment. All MS symptoms cause social problems. And this causes the MS victim to become irritable, depressed, and generally impossible to live with. There aren't many happy MS victims. There aren't many happy friends or family members either!

MS is confusing to people because they don't really understand it. Every doctor you talk to will give you a different cause and treatment. That's not surprising, because MS is a degenerative condition of the neurological system characterized by massive disagreement of opinion by any two people.

When you try to learn about MS, you quickly learn that not much information is available. It seems you don't find the information until you already know all about it. You start off with nothing more than the statement from your doctor that there is no known cause, no known cure, and it isn't fatal. If you become one of those who suffers from all the worst symptoms, you begin to wish it were fatal.

I don't have much respect for the medical profession's opinions of MS. They are more than happy to give you all the current information on the most recent theories. Did you pick up "current" and "most recent?" You see, as the high dollar research continues, the causes and possible treatments seem to continually change. With MS they are looking for a cure when they should be looking for the cause.

Let's define MS this way. There are two halves to the brain. The upper half does the thinking and the lower half controls motor functions in the body. From the base of the brain, nerves extend down the spinal column and out to the various muscles in the body. MS is simply a degeneration of the coating around the nerves. This coating is called the myelin sheath. The mind is not affected. The muscles are not affected, although they may appear to be. That is due to lack of use. There is no damage to the nerves. The nerves at the base of the brain are simply exposed where the degeneration of the myelin has occurred. This can prevent or misdirect the nerve impulse from traveling along its route to the muscles.

Even when I couldn't walk or feed myself, I felt like I could. I had normal sensation from the brain to the nerves. The impulse just didn't get to the muscles. I've caused my body to regenerate the myelin sheath where degeneration was. Like a cut finger, the body must do the healing.

When the myelin is missing, your nerve impulses become crossed and confused, and you lose the ability to control the muscle you're trying to use. Like a short in an electrical wire if it had no insulation to protect it. If the myelin is totally gone, the signal to your muscles may not go through at all. Doctors feel this myelin is replaced with scar tissue (sclerosis). I disagree. I feel the myelin is simply not there. I believe that if you help your body rebuild nutritionally, the myelin will grow back and protect the nerves as it should. This is what has happened to me. Through good nutrition, I have caused my body to regenerate the missing myelin. If the doctors are right and the myelin is replaced with scar tissue, the signals could never get through, could they? So how can doctors explain the remissions that MS people have? If you have a scar on your face, it's always there. It's not here today and gone tomorrow. Scars are permanent.

MS is a degenerative condition caused by poor nutrition and it can be corrected with proper nutrition. Controlling MS does not require high dollar research. It requires common sense!

We are so conditioned to accept what we are told by the medical profession that we seem to ignore the fact that they can't always be right. Much of medical training is financially subsidized by pharmaceutical firms who have prescription products to sell. They want our new doctors to be aware of these drugs. So medical schooling is a case of drug learning rather than nutritional learning. There is no profit in saying "This won't help," but there is profit to be made by saying, "This may help." I'm not saying the medical profession is totally money oriented, but no one will ever convince me a doctor would be a doctor if it brought him no income at all. And you don't earn any money by saying, "I can't help you."

Our local television station gave a statistic that over 80% of doctors office visits were for the common cold or the flu, two illnesses we know have no cure. Yet we go to them and get a wonderful prescription for something that won't help but does cost us money.

We will discuss this later, but right now let's return to the problem of MS. I think that maybe I'm not talking about the same sort of MS that the doctors talk of because there are some differences. With their MS, one day is bad, the next is good. One month you're down, the next month you're up. That's what mine was like until I became nutritionally aware. Once I started eating right, instead of attacks and remissions, I gained a control that is changed only by factors that I direct. I don't see this as a remission. I see it as a control. I can control it. I doesn't control me.

I am not cured of MS. I still have it. I simply have a method of controlling it through a few simple steps. I understand the medical attitude of it not being a provable statement for me to make. Yet I'm healthy. That's proof enough for me.

CHAPTER

6

Okay, you have MS or some other degenerative condition and you've been to your doctor and he has you on certain drugs and has enrolled you in a physical therapy program. Yet I'm suggesting that this is the wrong approach. I'm suggesting the use of nutrition for recovery. You're probably wondering what I base this on. Well, sit back because you won't believe this. I base it on facts we were all taught in grade school.

Do you remember your early health courses where you learned about the human body and had your first lessons on the four basic food groups? Facts were taught to us about nutritional needs and the importance of a balanced diet. We were taught that cells continually die in our body and are replaced by new cells through cell division. We were taught that we needed proper nutrition for this to happen. It's just like a house plant. If you don't water it and give it sunlight it will die. If your body does not get proper nutrition it won't be able to produce new cells at the same rate the old cells are dying. This is degeneration.

That's all I'm talking about with my MS control. I am

suggesting that we give our body the care we were taught to give it in grade school. Yet when I try to talk to people about my belief that good nutrition is necessary they don't seem to understand. I talk about the fact we do not get the nutrition we need from the food we eat and I am immediately labeled as crazy. People would rather listen to their doctor and the government talk about daily requirements of vitamins. I think those specialists are living in the past.

When speaking of nutrition, the medical field is using information that is no different than the information of 100 years ago. However, look at how our food has changed in the past 20 years much less 100 years. Nutritionally speaking, by the time today's food gets to our table, it is chemical garbage. From the very start our food takes a downward path in its trip to our tables. Our fruits and vegetables are sprayed with pesticides, treated with fertilizers and picked before they are ripe. Then they are shipped across the country and chemically ripened by your food supplier. If you buy food in a fresh, raw state, you are buying food that has been subjected to several chemicals that are clearly labeled as dangerous for human consumption. Do they think you buy food just to look at it?

To make things more interesting, look at the meat products we eat. Chicken comes to our table without the birds ever seeing the sun. Our meat products come to us after having been raised with hormones, chemicals and tranquilizers. We are eating that!

Then we make it worse on our own by eating food from the fifth food group that the last generation has developed, junk food. Fast food that starts with chemically grown produce and meat that is canned, frozen or dried, and treated with more chemicals to preserve it. Then it sits under a heat lamp waiting for us to buy it. How can we believe this is good for us?

How can you expect the cells in your body to divide and grow if you are feeding it garbage like this? Yet because we're too lazy to prepare our own food and because we don't all have the means of growing our own food, we are trapped by the system. What can you do to change it though? I'm afraid we will never change the commercial way of growing food. But I'll argue to the end with those specialists and professionals who claim we are still getting the same nutritional value. They say that the new processes can be countered by chemically adding vitamins. The problem is too many chemicals already. I don't want chemical vitamins added to it, not when a chemical vitamin can't compare to nature's own system.

So we sit back and let others tell us what we need. Have you ever looked at the back of a vitamin bottle? They give you the RDA (recommended daily allowance) as established by the government. It will usually show the dosage as being suitable for anyone over four or six years of age. I can't believe that a six-year-old sitting in first grade has the same nutritional need as a 200 pound grown man who smokes, drinks and works as a bricklayer. Even doctors tell you that stress robs your body of certain vitamins, that smoking robs you of vitamin C and that altitude robs you of zinc. Yet you are supposed to believe that everyone needs the same amount of all vitamins. If that seems logical to you, you may as well close this book. Yet we accept the statement from all those professionals that a normal food diet, with the possible addition of a chemical multi-vitamin, is sufficient for good health. That must be why we have no sick people, right?

I am suggesting our best hope for good health is to try to stick to fresh organically grown foods as much as possible and back it up with good food supplements. Notice I did not say vitamins. I said food supplements. I'm referring to vitamins in tablet or capsule form that come from whole food sources rather than some chemist's test tube. It doesn't make them a perfect supplement just better than the chemical form. Even supplements from whole food sources can't be perfect because the original food has been subjected to the chemicals in our water supply and the pollutants in our air. But it's the best there presently is. Our food supply is going to get worse if we don't do something to change it.

Having MS, you need to make these changes in your diet and even some more radical ones if your condition is bad. You need to rebuild your body. We'll talk more about nutrition later.

CHAPTER

7

Obviously this book is headed in a particular direction. At some point I will start talking about what I am doing and why you should do it as well. Before we do that, let's look at other treatments and examine why we choose to use them.

From our youngest years we are taught to see our physician when we are ill. That statement is tossed at us on every bottle of pills we buy. Our advertising force also advises us to see our doctor when in doubt. When you buy cold tablets (which aren't going to cure anything), the bottle directs you to consult a physician if the medication causes the listed side effects. When the side effects occur, you go to your doctor, and he tells you to stop taking the remedy. Why do you need a doctor to tell you that? When the medicine causes problems, can't you use your own reasoning to decide you shouldn't take it? After all, your mind works cheaper than an office call to your doctor.

We've become guilty of abusing the "consult your physician" statement. When we we're taught to see our doctor for problems, I believe they originally were referring to things like broken bones, severe cuts, ruptured appendix, injuries needing surgery

same batch of hair by several different companies and have several different results. Even if hair analysis were accurate in its test method it would only tell you what is in the hair shaft itself. That is determined by your shampoo, the air around you, the amount of sun you get, and the nutrients supplied by your body. Blood tests are a bit better. At least they can get an accurate test result of what your blood has in it. Does that tell you what you need? Only your body can tell you what it needs. Everyone is different.

Maybe you should decide on chiropractic care. Maybe it will help and maybe you'll get some relief. Possibly though, you'll find one of those chiropractors who wants you to come back for a weekly tune up so you can pay him again and again. It seems to be another side of the medical profession going astray. Twenty years ago, a chiropractic treatment was supposed to correct your problem. Today it's supposed to get you by until the next tune-up. Totally illogical!

How about kinesiology? Why not? We all have money to burn, right? And it will relax you. It's more fun to pay $40 for a relaxing massage than to have your spouse do it, right?

Snake venom? Gold injections? Hyperbaric oxygenation? Chemotherapy? And on and on and on. Why not? After all, if we can't believe the doctor, we have to believe someone, right? We have to have someone telling us what to do.

Why not take vitamins? Lots of people selling vitamins will tell you that's all you need. Even some people selling the brand of supplements I use myself have the mistaken notion that vitamins alone can cure you.

We could go to a psychiatrist and be told it's all in our head. That's probably closest to the truth of the entire matter.

There are lots of treatments we can spend our money on to attempt a health cure. But if everyone agrees that MS is a degeneration of myelin, how can they believe any of these treatments will help. We need something that will cause rebuilding not just something designed to halt the degeneration. I realize we get desperate and become willing to try anything. I did it myself. But I also reached a point where I realized that I had to help myself. I developed a firm belief that one can control, not just treat, many of the "illnesses" that occur.

When we step away from the medical field and look for other means of help, we have a tendency to grab some other treatment, silly or not. We give the person who convinced us of its value the same trust and lack of personal concern we gave the doctor. We're insulting our own intelligence.

In the remainder of this book, I am going to tell you what I did to regain my health. I will be just like the doctors, the chiropractors, the experimenting scientists, the vitamin sellers and all the others. I will try to convince you to try what I believe will work. There are some differences between their ways and mine though. Mine has actually worked. But I honestly don't think it will work for everyone.

CHAPTER

8

That's a crazy statement to make to those of you who are used to someone telling you to follow their program and all will be well. But it's the absolute truth. I have never told anyone that this will absolutely, positively cure them. The method I use will never cure MS or anything else. It will control it though. And in a world that has no cure or treatment for MS, that's good enough for me. I've said before and will say again, I sincerely believe that the method I use will work for anyone who lets it work. That sounds a bit confusing, so let's clear the matter up by discussing the first control I use to keep myself healthy which is attitude.

You can read many successful health stories about cancer victims, diabetics, accident victims, and others talking about the methods those people used. Exercise, diet, vitamins, and other methods have separately been used very successfully. But what made it work? Professionals are finally beginning to realize that the individual's attitude toward their health problem has much to do with the cure even with medical treatments. I recently heard a pharmaceutical firm spokesman say that the public buys medicine in capsule form because they think it is more potent. He added to his statement by saying that if people believe capsules work better, they actually do! He was saying that the effectiveness of medication is determined partly by your attitude toward it.

Those people who truly want to get better and are willing to do everything they can to succeed seem to have better results than those who leave it to their doctor or therapist to help them. Success requires a belief in success. You control your own destiny.

I don't have much sympathy for those who can't get or don't have the proper attitude to succeed in their battle. I think some people are happy with their bad health, and I don't have the time to waste on them. I surround myself with those who have the desire to be healthy.

You see, this little control I use is rather unique. No one can give it to you. No doctor can prescribe it. No friends or family can make you do it. Spending an hour talking to me will not make it work for you. It's something you have to want to do all by yourself. No one can make you feel that this will work. It's impossible for someone to instill the solid belief that "this is it" in you. You have to reach that point all by yourself. You alone, are responsible for your health, your body, and yourself. Just you!

I get calls all the time from people who want to talk about my present health and how they can get there also. If they read about my method and still need proof or assurance it will work it probably won't! They don't have faith and a desire for good health. They are only wanting me to tell them it will work. They must have that belief by themselves. They come to me with the standard misconceptions of their problem and try to trade it off for a belief in my opinions. For success, it must be their own personal belief.

If you start on the program I use and say, "My doctor tells me this won't work," it won't! If you say, "I don't know if it will work, but I'll try," it won't work! If you say, "I wish, I hope, I'll try," it won't work! You must be totally convinced and committed to the effort. It isn't easy. It's big changes in lifestyle. It makes others think you've flipped out. It has family grumbling about the cost, even though it's cheaper than most medical treatments.

Knowing you can recover is very important. You must be willing to make changes. You must be ready to place your trust in yourself.

The person with MS seems to have five problems in attitude. They are family, friends, doctors, the local MS support chapter, and their own self. That's something, huh? How can you stay away from everyone you know and not do any thinking about yourself either? Impossible? Not at all! What makes these people into problems? Let's look at that.

Family and friends create the same problem. They feel sorry for you. They feel sorry for those around you. They try to do everything they can to help you. They spoil you. They feel so sorry for you that you start feeling sorry for yourself. You probably didn't need any help with that anyway. Being told you have MS makes you feel sorry all by yourself. How can you stop their honest and sincere efforts to help you? Do you have to actually tell them to leave you alone and let you do it your way? *Yes!*

I know that not everyone will try to kill you with kindness. But I know from my own experience that it was impossible for my mother to watch me struggle with my coat. My family couldn't leave me on the ground when I fell. They couldn't bear to see my need for extra time to complete simple tasks. They *had* to help. They loved me. They couldn't stand to see me take supplements that choked me when the doctor had a simple injection that might help. They couldn't stand to see me passing up the holiday candies and cakes, because they knew how much I enjoyed the taste of those goodies. They wanted the best for me.

When I met my wife, she also wanted the best for me. She cooked me foods that were right, she laughed at me and made me mad so I worked myself harder. She noticed the things that were improving and she criticized my faults. She treated me like a regular person. That is the sort of person you need to surround yourself with as you work toward better health. Let the ones with sympathy donate their time to help those who need sympathy and comfort. Tell them to stop being so solicitous. Move away if you have to. Make the best of your situation. Don't shut yourself up. Listen to motivational tapes on any subject. If you don't start with the right attitude, brainwash yourself to develop it!

What about the doctors and the local MS chapter? They want to help also, right? Of course they do! But they are giving

you more of the same. It's a big pity party. You can go to MS meetings and find a group who want to talk about how bad it was this week or how nice their new electric wheelchair is. These people have made the decision to find those who will be sympathetic to their problems and who will work at making it easier for them. You can't do those things and expect a diet change to make you healthy again. Feeling sorry for yourself or trying to make things easier is not the right way.

And yourself? How can you be hurting yourself? If you feel sorry for yourself, you are hurting yourself. If you are looking for ways to make your life easier, you are hurting yourself. If you are listening to everyone's sympathy, you are hurting yourself. It's really quite simple. If you say to yourself, "I can't do that anymore," you are hurting yourself. If you say, "I've got to find a way to do that again," you'll probably find it.

I hurt myself greatly by saying, I'll never get in a wheelchair." I was acknowledging the reality of the wheelchair. I should have been telling myself, I need to learn how to walk again. I believe you need to convince yourself that "worse" does not exist, to the point that it doesn't even enter your thoughts.

When speaking of attitude, I can't help but remember one lady with MS who had a very loving husband. As her health started downward, he did everything in his power to help her. He brought her chocolates, he went shopping for knitting supplies to keep her busy, and he added a new bedroom onto their home that had floor-to-ceiling windows to entertain her when she finally became bedridden. To prepare for the grim future, this bedroom also had an I-beam running across the ceiling that would enable him to use a sling hoist to get her from bed to bath. It was a dream home for a permanently disabled person. In my opinion, it was a nightmare for an MS person. How did he expect her to try to do things for herself when he was so lovingly preventing her from doing anything at all? He did the cooking, the cleaning, and ran to get her anything she wanted. She sat all day in her chair and acted like a queen. Who wouldn't? Yet they couldn't understand when I said I didn't think anything I was doing could help her.

This is a direct example of killing with kindness. How much better it would have been if his support had been a healthier, helpful type. I admired the love he had for her but I left there feeling bad about the way he expressed that love.

It isn't always the family that hurts us, though. Sometimes we do it all by ourselves. We become our own worst enemy.

One medical doctor I knew was quite impressed with my recovery. He had known me when I was at my worst health and was quite delighted to see me in my present good health. He wasn't sure that my program of nutrition was responsible, but he acknowledged that the treatments he had offered hadn't given such good results. Because of this, he started suggesting to his MS patients that they visit with me. He didn't endorse my methods he simply encouraged his patients to explore my theories and consider the use of them. He wrote prescriptions for them to defray the cost of supplements through the use of insurance. He had their dieticians visit with me to insure these patients were eating the foods that I ate. He did everything he could to help his patients. He was a very special doctor who was willing to admit he didn't have all the answers.

I remember the first girl that called me. Because he suggested this might help, she decided to try it. Her insurance paid for the supplements covered by his prescription. A local charity cooked her meals, delivered them, and fed them to her. Another group helped her with exercise and shopping. She stayed with it for two weeks and then called me again.

She said it wasn't helping. She felt she had given it a fair chance. She felt that sugar wasn't hurting her. She missed eating pizza and was convinced that something tasting so good couldn't possibly be bad for her. She quit! You see, she didn't want to be healthy again. The only people who wanted good health for her were her doctor, the volunteers and me. She was very happy being waited on. She enjoyed lying in bed until someone got her up and dressed her. It's hard to walk away from someone like that and leave them alone, but it's the only thing you can do. The best help you can give someone with MS is to support them in their own beliefs. Even if it means doing nothing.

This is why attitude is hard to understand. Many times the family wants to help more than the situation calls for. Some people are totally content sitting in a wheelchair and being waited on all the time. Nothing will help them. There are also those who have a super attitude. They will accomplish the impossible.

I remember when a young couple came to my home. She had MS, and it took her about ten minutes to get from the car into the house using a cane. She suffered from blindness in one eye and truly bad coordination problems. They wanted to know about what I was doing and we visited for an hour or more. She was very excited about all of it, convinced that it would work for her, and left my home telling me she was so happy that she would be healthy again. Four days later I received a call from her husband. Her sight had returned, the tremors were gone, and she was jogging! He said he hadn't expected nutrition to change things so fast. I had a hard time convincing him that nothing I had suggested would work that fast. I honestly believe she was capable and able to do those things before she visited with me. Nutrition does not work that fast. I think she had been so convinced by everyone she would have problems that she mentally willed herself into bad health. Her visit with me had simply reversed those thoughts and made her aware that she could improve.

To follow up on this, they continued to read about nutrition and attitude. They mentioned it to their doctor who told them she would hurt herself taking all those supplements. On the advice of her doctor, she stopped the use of supplements and diet change. Her health reverted to its former poor condition, but she was content because she was doing what the doctor wanted her to do.

I have spoken with several people who refused my help because they wanted to keep their MS a secret. One person I know was so embarrassed by the thought of MS, that she always carried a drink at home and when she was away she splashed bourbon on herself so people would think her staggering walk was from being drunk! Another lady hadn't even told her husband or children that she had MS. I don't know how she dealt with it when the symptoms got worse and hiding it became impossible.

I could go on with example after example of different attitudes. Each person seems to have their own way of handling life. But there are some basic matters that affect all of us with MS.

We all have a tendency to let the things we hear affect our way of thinking. We hear that MS is fatal. It's not! I've heard people refer to the brain damage caused by MS. That isn't true. There is nothing wrong with the mind. You suffer so much mental anguish with MS that it becomes easy to convince yourself there is something wrong mentally. And there is, it's called frustration, not brain damage.

I received a call one day from a lady with MS who was preparing to take her life. She said she couldn't live with the personality change it caused. As we visited, she talked about how mad she was at everyone and how it had led to a divorce. It was making it difficult for her own parents to be around her. She found it hard to believe that she was experiencing a normal reaction to MS. I told her I thought her anger was good as long as she recognized that she was mad about the MS and not mad at her family. I get upset that MS people aren't told that anger is normal. Why not use that anger to fight the disease instead of using it to fight with those you love? It's easy to use anger properly if you know that it's okay to have that anger.

An entire book could be written about attitude. As a matter of fact, there are many books about attitude. Perhaps they aren't dealing specifically with your problem, but that isn't important. What's important is that you recognize the value of attitude in your health.

As it states at the start of this book, I am not a doctor. I can't tell anyone what to do. I can share with you what I have done for myself. I feel you are passing up a great opportunity if you don't do this for yourself. You have everything to gain and nothing to lose. When I see people quit because they don't get immediate results, it makes me mad. It took me five years but it was sure worth it.

When I spoke earlier about this method not working for everyone, I was referring to the importance of attitude. I've heard a bad attitude being compared to a flat tire. You can't go anywhere until you change it. I sincerely believe you can control your destiny largely through attitude. It isn't all of it, but it's most of it.

CHAPTER

9

If an attitude isn't all of it, then what else did I do? After working on the health of my mind, I began working on the health of my body. A very important part of recovery is accomplished through rest and adequate exercise.

Those of us with MS seem to tire easily. We need more rest than other people need. Don't let others make you feel guilty about that. When you are tired, stop! If you are out for a walk and reach a point of exhaustion, sit down in someone's yard and rest a while. Don't concern yourself with how it looks. A friend of mine had trouble with a stumbling, staggering gait. It embarrassed her to see people staring at her. She didn't let that stop her from the daily walking she needed though. She had a T-shirt made that said, "I'm not drunk! I always walk this way." After that when she went for a walk, she wore her T-shirt and felt more confident. She dealt with it.

Don't let others tell you how much rest you need. You are the only one who knows when to quit. Work at your own pace. Believe in yourself.

Fatigue was probably my last symptom of MS to leave me. I

still suffer from it. My wife called me Captain Sofa. I will never put myself in a position where I can't control the amount of rest I get. It's very important for my health to be rested and relaxed. There are times when I am accused of just being a lazy person. Sometimes maybe I am! But I have MS. What good is it if I can't use it for an occasional chance to get out of the yard work?

And exercise? I have a strange attitude toward that also. My policy is "Do what you can." I don't think any therapist could possibly know what my body requires in exercise. I don't think anyone can tell me when to stop or when to continue. I am not training for the Olympics. I do not need to push myself to super human limits. I simply need to exercise my body in an effort to rebuild muscle tissue. You must be willing to physically work yourself but you don't have to turn into Superman to be healthy. Use a combination of walking, bicycling, sit-ups, or whatever you are comfortable with. When I got out of the wheelchair, I needed more strength in my legs. I used my arm strength to help me do deep knee bends and as my legs became stronger, I used more leg movement and less arm movement.

The important thing to remember is that you must do all of the steps to recover your health. You cannot expect a good attitude to do it alone. You must be willing to work your physical body to its limit and then give it the necessary rest.

And that's about all there is to say regarding rest and exercise. Do what you can and rest when you must.

CHAPTER

10

E arlier I talked about the need for proper nutrition. We need to now take that a step further and discuss the additional changes that are used by many to control MS. When I first started searching for answers to MS, separate from the medical society's opinions, I had a hard time finding information. Perhaps it was because I wasn't specifically looking for a nutritional answer.

We must all admit that good nutrition is important. We need to realize that modern food is not filling our nutritional needs. To make matters worse, MS people seem to have allergies to specific foods. I am not suggesting extensive allergy testing. I think that is one more effort on our part to put the responsibility of our health onto someone else's shoulders. I choose to use the findings of other MS people who treated themselves and use the things that worked for them. I know that they also worked for me. Perhaps I didn't need to eliminate all the foods that I did, but with the success I had, I'm not going to back up and try a different method.

As I start with the diet changes I made, please remember I

am simply relating to you what I, myself, did. Whether or not you choose to do it is your own decision. Don't let me or anyone else decide that for you.

The first and biggest change in my diet was eliminating sugar. I am not a chemist or food expert. I do not know the chemical capabilities of sugar. I only know that once I eliminated sugar from my diet, I could see a noticeable change in my tremors. I switched to honey for a sweetener. I used artificial sweeteners. I realize there is a debate as to the cancer causing properties of those, but I was trying to get rid of my MS problems, and I wasn't going to worry about a condition I didn't even have. Getting refined sugar out of my diet was more important to me at the time. I do not claim to know why sugar causes such problems for me or others. The debate over sugar will go on for many years. Sugar has been linked to crime levels, children's behavioral problems, hyperactivity, and many other issues. For everyone who says it is a problem, there is someone else stating that it is not! You have to draw your own conclusions. I chose to eliminate it because I felt better without it. This did not happen the first day I went without sugar. I wasn't even aware of the difference until I had been off sugar for a few months and then had the experience of eating food with sugar in it.

Most people will change their food habits and three days later return to the old ways because they notice no changes. Believe me, bad health does not happen overnight. It took a lot of years of poor eating to cause the problems. You can't expect good eating habits to immediately correct them. You must be willing to give it time. I had nothing but time!

When I read of the man in England who used diet change to recover from MS, the article mentioned leaving glutens out of your diet because they had the same effect as sugar. In the spirit of "I'll try anything," I added glutens to my list of food to avoid. Glutens are wheat, rye, oats, barley and buckwheat. This eliminated breads, breakfast cereals, canned soups, cakes, cookies and such from my diet. That was okay because by avoiding sugar I had already removed canned vegetables, soft drinks, and most prepared foods.

The last food I eliminated was animal fat. This seemed to be viewed as a good step by everyone out there. At least this didn't have the continual debate that sugar seemed to cause in everyone. I did nothing fancy to eliminate animal fat. I simply quit eating red meat and switched to chicken or fish. I started using low fat milk, diet margarines, cut back on my intake of cheeses, switched to sunflower oil for cooking and eliminated as much fried food as possible.

I've never understood the problems people have in changing their diet. I never viewed any of this as extreme or impossible. I still ate pizza but it simply had a few changes in it. Like the gluten free rice crust which is tastier than a standard flour crust.

The diet change is not radical. I do not shop in specialty health food stores. The foods I need to buy are right in the grocery store. I just had to spend my first few weeks learning to read labels and remembering what brands were all right for my body.

I do not like to mention name brands. I'm not trying to knock any food item and it would appear that I was if I started saying what I consider safe or unsafe. Simply read labels. As an example, there are several brands of ketchup on the store shelves. In the ingredient list, some are made using sugar and others are made using corn syrup. Use the brands made with corn syrup. Look for the cheaper products in canned vegetables that are canned without the expense of sugar. Use fresh or frozen foods as much as possible.

Simply use common sense and caution. I do what feels right for my own body. I don't let someone else tell me what I should eat. Please remember that. When you start to feel that you have to do just what I did, remember that I am saying you should do what feels right for you. If sitting in a wheelchair eating candy feels right for you then do it! If you feel better by eating good and working at improvement, then do it. Don't let anyone force you into some treatment you're not happy using.

I am always asked to give particulars on my diet such as sample meals. People want me to tell them what to eat for each meal. Those are the people who shouldn't even try my approach. They have an attitude problem. They want me to take the place of their doctor or therapist. No thank you! If you don't have enough ambition to read food labels, you don't have enough ambition to help yourself. I will give some sample meals in a later chapter, but it is done to give a general idea of my diet. It is not a regiment to be followed for a "cure."

Why am I so convinced that eliminating these foods has helped? How do I know it's not just a remission? These are honest questions that have a very simple answer.

When I first used a combination of diet change and

supplements, I felt better but was not doing noticeably better. As my body gradually rebuilt itself, I started showing improvement in all areas. When I was away from home traveling and had to rely on restaurant meals, I tried to be careful about what I ate. I didn't have the final control on whether the orange juice was a concentrate or fresh. I didn't know if the hash browns were fresh or frozen. Most brands of frozen potatoes have added sugar for that golden brown appearance. When I ate foods that I wasn't totally sure of, my health slowly deteriorated.

Three days of eating away from home would put me right back down. I would have to go back on an extremely strict sugar free, gluten free diet. In a few days I would be okay again. It was noticeable that I could control my problems. This was my own personal proof that it was not a remission. It did what I caused it to do. It wasn't just a random MS problem.

As my health got better and better, I did become more lax about my diet. But, I could feel when I had overstepped my limits and knew when to get tough with myself and eat right.

Even two years after I appeared to be healthy, a simple sugared soft drink would cause a visible tremor in my left eye that was unnoticed by me but very apparent to those looking at me. Presently, that does not occur. I seem to have rebuilt my body to a point where it can stand more abuse than before. That is probably the whole key to the matter. We all abuse our bodies. We simply need to find our abuse limit.

At this point in my health, I do have a more normal diet than I did while I was trying to rebuild myself. I do occasionally eat sugared items. I have an occasional steak or hamburger. I do socially consume alcoholic beverages. But I can feel when I have overstepped my limits. I can tell when to straighten up and eat right. I have learned to pay attention to my body and do what feels right. I have not expected anyone else to control what happens to me.

CHAPTER

11

When you make a diet change as I have done, you cause other things to happen. Many of the foods I eliminated have necessary, healthy nutrients in them. For example, the glutens are a great source of the B vitamins. But I don't eat glutens. The dairy products, wheat products, the red meat products and other foods all have good nutrients in them that my personal diet omits. So I had to find a way of getting the nutrients without eating those foods. My supposedly healthy diet wasn't worth much if I suffered from a lack of nutrition. So I needed to supplement my diet with those missing nutrients. This is why I take food supplements.

Let's remember that a vitamin is a product chemically produced that has the properties of the vitamin it is supposed to be. A food supplement is a product resulting from the extraction of nutrients from a whole food source. A food supplement is the food without the bulk.

There are many brands of vitamins and supplements available. I am not promoting the product brand I use because many would see it as a commercial effort. I will advise you to be wary of the label "Natural Vitamin." *Everything* is natural. Plastic bags are natural. Everything comes from nature. Even chemicals come from nature. Therefore, every vitamin is natural. Look for a product that states it comes from a whole food source. Realize that a whole food source supplement can't be compressed into a small tablet that can be taken once a day. Due to the fact that you will be consuming the nutrients of whole foods, you will probably find that supplement use will require the consumption of many tablets.

I think this is what gets the medical profession so upset. They think that if you are taking 60 tablets a day, you must surely be taking too much. Yet these same doctors wouldn't be at all upset if you ate ten carrots a day or seven oranges a day. They don't realize that's precisely what you are eating with your supplements. They are going on their trained theory that when you put a chemical vitamin into the body, the body has it whether it needs it or not. They don't understand that a food supplement is just like a food. If your body doesn't need it, it will simply reject what it doesn't need.

It is correct to assume then that you will be wasting some of your supplement consumption. Some of that will pass straight through you and be discarded in your body waste. In other words, you will flush a lot of it right down the toilet. When I first started taking supplements I was definitely taking too much. I didn't know how much to take and I wanted to make sure I had enough. My urine almost glowed in the dark!

As my body became used to the addition of supplements, it started telling me what to take. I just had to watch and learn.

When my urine was overly bright, I knew I was wasting the B and C vitamins. When I got droopy, I knew I needed more zinc. I didn't have to study any book or become a vitamin expert to know this. I just started learning from what was happening to my body. You see, everyone is different. Everyone has different needs. But if everyone would pay more attention to their body, they would be surprised at what they would learn.

When someone tells me they could never learn to do this, I think they are forgetting something. They already listen to their body to tell them when to eat or sleep. They let their body tell them when to go to the bathroom. They know when the body says it's hot. They put a coat on when the body tells them it's cold. Why don't they think they can hear it telling them what it needs nutritionally? They just need to listen.

I spent years taking the products that doctors suggested. I just kept getting worse. When I started taking what my body suggested, I improved. That's all I need to know about supplements! Let me show you the difference.

The doctors gave me these drugs between 1971 and 1976:

Prednisone

Stelazine

ACTHIV

Dexedrine

Acthar Gel

Lioresal

Ritalin

Arnica Kneipp

Larodopa

Clonopin

Valium

Depo Provera

Sinemet

Depo Testosterone Extradiol

Tofranil

Arnica Plantaplex

Dantrium

Meprobamate

Serax

Parlodel Bromocriptine

Symmetrel

I presently take these supplements:

Protein

B-Complex

Herbal Laxative

Magnesium

Alfalfa

Calcium

Lecithin

Vitamin C

Vitamin E

Zinc

Beta Carotene

Multi-Vitamin

Which list of products would you rather consume?

I feel that all of this is necessary for my body's health. There is no way I would quit taking the supplements or get off the diet. It's just too much fun living a full life. When someone tells me I'm on a crazy, difficult diet and that supplements are too costly, I think back to those years in the wheelchair. If this is what crazy and costly does, then give me more.

I'm not a doctor. I don't know what everyone needs. I don't even know what I need, but my body knows. I give it the best foods I possibly can, and I give it a lot of supplements. I let it use what it needs. I don't worry about taking too much since it's from a whole food source. Even when I was taking almost 200 tablets a day of food supplements, I was not taking mega-doses of vitamins.

CHAPTER

12

When I tell people I eat no glutens, little animal fat and no sugar, they always ask "what do you eat?" Actually I have a very good diet and a fun selection of foods. It took a bit longer in the grocery store at first. Reading labels and looking for sugar free items. It also required that my wife spend some time learning how to substitute honey and rice flour into regular recipes. The result of that work was a daily plan of meals that was very tasty. I'm not a nutritionist. I'm simply an MS person who found something that works for me. I really feel that everyone has different needs. But even doctors are impressed with my diet.

In the interest of showing you a sample of my diet, let me give you the following week's menu. The nicest thing about my present diet is that I eat more different foods than I did before. I eat foods that taste good. I eat foods that are good for me. It wasn't hard to change. Please realize that the diet isn't 100% cruel, there are times I sneak something extra into my diet. In other words, nothing's perfect!

Some of the foods listed will appear to be incompatible

with my diet. A further check in the recipe section will show you how these foods are made safe for me. Many standard recipes can be used by simply changing product brands or the sweetener used.

With my meals I drink fresh juices, low fat milk, coffee, iced tea, hot tea or water. I also drink soft drinks or generic brands that are sweetened with corn syrup.

MONDAY

Breakfast
Pancakes, maple syrup, poached egg, fresh juice
Lunch
Turkey sandwich, potato chips, fresh fruit
Dinner
Pizza, salad, and garlic toast

TUESDAY

Breakfast
Poached egg, toast and hash browns
Lunch
Chicken or turkey frank with French fries and fresh fruit
Dinner
Spicy chicken breasts, corn on the cob and scalloped Potatoes Au Gratin

WEDNESDAY

Breakfast

Omelet, rice patty toasted, fruit

Lunch

Salad and soup

Dinner

Cheesy rice casserole, tossed salad, apple muffins

THURSDAY

Breakfast

Puffed rice cereal with low fat milk, grapefruit, toast

Lunch

Tuna sandwich on rice bread and potato chips

Dinner

Baked or broiled fish, peas and biscuits

FRIDAY

Breakfast

Poached eggs, bacon strips and toast

Lunch

Hamburger patty, corn and bread

Dinner

Baked chicken, baked potato, green beans and banana bread

SATURDAY

Breakfast
Fresh fruit, toast and juice
Lunch
Leftover pizza with a salad
Dinner
Mexican casserole with salad and corn bread

SUNDAY

Breakfast
French toast and eggs
Lunch
Chicken salad sandwich with a vegetable and fruit
Dinner
Fried chicken, corn and mashed potatoes with gravy

DESSERTS

Sponge cake, jelly rolls, banana cream delight, apple muffins, pineapple pudding, chiffon cake, peanut butter squares, cake with frosting, nut cookies, honey peanut butter candy and banana bread.

As you can tell, it appears to be a basic, normal diet. There are changes though. Pancakes are made with rice flour. All breads are bought in the local stores, gluten free. Many brands of potato chips and such are processed without added chemicals.

Fried foods are occasionally okay for me if they are cooked in sunflower oil. Eating bacon is possible if I use the soy product bacon strips.

Regardless of attitude, rest and exercise being so important, it still relates to the two big changes of diet and supplements. Fortunately, with a little work, we made the diet a small change that worked good as healthy food for the whole family. I must admit that the rest of the family doesn't like gluten free rice bread. But we can still eat the same sandwiches and such. I use my bread and they use theirs.

It is still difficult to eat meals in restaurants. I have no way of knowing the source of their foods. I can't tell if it's fresh or frozen potatoes. I don't know if it's fresh juice or concentrate. I can eat lots of vegetables and fruits on my own and save the restaurant dining for special times. And of course, now that I'm healthy again, I seem to be able to endure those unsure meals as long as I back it up with good meals at home.

CHAPTER

13

I t was easy for us to adapt this diet and way of cooking into our family eating habits. We shop for brands of canned goods that do not contain sugar or flour. Some brands of vegetables are processed with sugar and others will be sugar free. We did not have to go into dietetic foods much at all. It was usually just a matter of watching labels and brands. We use fresh or frozen fruit and vegetables as much as possible. Buying or growing back yard fresh foods gives us produce that has more vitamins remaining in them. Their food value isn't lost through shipping and sitting in warehouses and grocery stores. It gives the added advantage of less chemicals used in the growth of the food. The following recipes all use standard canned goods or fresh items.

Most standard recipes using flour can be made using rice flour rather than wheat flour. Brown rice flour will result in a better, less chalky tasting recipe. In cakes and cookies, cooling the batter or dough before baking will result in a finished product that is not so crumbly or apt to fall apart. There is a definite difference in taste between wheat and rice flour. Your individual taste will tell you which foods you can enjoy using rice flour. They aren't all bad!

In recipes that call for sugar, the general rule is to reduce the amount of liquid 1/4 cup for each cup of honey used. Honey may be substituted for sugar cup for cup. When honey is substituted in baked goods, add 1/2 teaspoon of baking soda to the recipe for every cup of honey used and bake at a lower temperature. Honey can also be used in any cold drink, but I have found it does not keep well. With some cold drinks, the following day it will taste bitterly spoiled. I mix only what I will drink in one day.

In most baked recipes, honey will not affect the taste any differently than sugar. I also use maple syrup and fructose sweeteners.

The following recipes are just an example of what is possible. There are thousands of recipes that are just fine or can be easily changed. All of my recipes were a result of taking the foods I enjoyed eating and making small changes that kept them healthy for me.

MEXICAN CASSEROLE

1 lb. hamburger
1 tsp. chili powder
1/4 cup chopped onion
1 can refried beans
8 corn tortillas
1 cup sour cream
2 cups grated cheddar cheese
Hot sauce
2 (15 oz) cans tomato sauce
3 crushed, dried red peppers

Brown hamburger, drain and add onion. Season as desired and add chili powder. Stir in refried beans. Layer in a 13 x 9 baking dish in the following order: sauce, tortillas, 1/2 of the meat mixture, sour cream, sauce, tortillas, sauce, rest of the meat mixture, cheese, tortillas, sauce and cheese. Bake at 350 for 40 minutes. Watch canned goods for those processed without sugar.

CHEESY RICE CASSEROLE

1 beaten egg
1 chopped onion
1/2 cup grated cheese
1 cup milk
2 cups cooked brown rice
1/2 tablespoon oil

Use oil to grease casserole dish. Mix all ingredients together. Put in casserole and bake at 350 until set.

PIZZA HOT DISH

1 lb. hamburger
1/4 cup chopped onion
1 cup tomato sauce
1/2 lb. noodles or rice
1 cup mushrooms
1/2 lb. grated Mozzarella cheese
1/2 teaspoon garlic salt
1/2 teaspoon salt
1/4 teaspoon pepper

Brown hamburger and onion, drain fat. Add tomato sauce and seasonings; simmer 30 minutes. Cook noodles. Combine meat mixture and noodles with mushrooms. Put into 8 x 10 baking dish and cover with cheese. Bake at 325 for 25 minutes.

Meatloaf

1 lb. ground beef
1 egg
1/2 cup cooked rice
1/2 cup powdered milk
1 chopped onion
1 teaspoon salt
1/2 cup water
1 cup tomatoes

Blend all ingredients together. Put in greased loaf pan. Bake at 350 for 1 hour.

Scalloped Potatoes Au Gratin

4 potatoes, peeled and thinly sliced
3 tablespoons rice flour or potato starch flour
1 teaspoon salt
1/2 small diced onion
1 cup grated cheddar cheese
1 cup scalded milk
2 tablespoons butter

Arrange half of the potatoes in bottom of greased 8 inch casserole dish. Combine flour and salt, sprinkle half of it over potatoes. Spread half of the cheese over this. Repeat layers of potatoes, flour and cheese. Pour hot milk over this and dot with butter. Cook uncovered in microwave oven 12 to 14 minutes until potatoes are tender, or bake at 350 in covered dish in conventional oven until tender. Serves 4.

Pancakes

1 cup soya flour
2 tablespoons melted butter
2 teaspoons baking powder
1 cup yellow cornmeal
1/2 teaspoon salt
1 3/4 cup of milk
2 eggs

Beat eggs well. Add all other ingredients and beat well. Fry on heavy griddle.

Spicy Chicken Breasts

4 chicken breasts (remove skin)
2 large tomatoes (mash or put in blender)
1/2 teaspoon basil
1/2 teaspoon oregano
1/2 teaspoon chili powder
Onion and garlic powder to taste

Put chicken flesh side up in casserole dish. Mix other ingredients together and pour over chicken. Bake covered at 350 for one hour or until done.

Tossed Salad

Chopped lettuce
Chopped dill pickle
1 pkg. frozen peas
2 cups diet mayonnaise
Shredded onion
Bacon Bits
Shredded cheese

Using a 9 x 12 layer pan, layer lettuce and frozen peas. Mix onion, pickle and mayonnaise; cover top of layers with this. Sprinkle cheese and bacon bits on top. Let set overnight.

Gravy

Prepare as you normally would substituting rice flour for wheat flour. There is really no difference in taste or texture.

Sponge Cake

1 cup honey

1 cup potato starch

1/4 teaspoon salt

1 teaspoon lemon juice

6 egg yolks

2 teaspoons baking powder

3 tablespoons water

6 egg whites

Beat egg yolks, gradually add honey while beating. Sift dry ingredients together and add to yolks. Add water and flavoring. Beat thoroughly. Beat egg whites until stiff and fold into cake mixture. Pour batter into a tube pan and bake at 300 for one hour.

Jelly Roll

Prepare above recipe for Sponge Cake as indicated. Bake on a cookie sheet with sides for 20 minutes. Line sheet with waxed paper. Remove at once, spread with jelly and roll while warm. Use jelly processed with honey rather than sugar.

FRIED CHICKEN

Remove skin from chicken pieces. Roll the chicken in rice flour to coat well. Cover bottom of skillet with sunflower oil. Cook covered over medium low heat for 20 minutes. Do not remove lid before 20 minutes. Turn pieces over and cook covered 20 minutes on the other side. Season to taste and serve.

BANANA CREAM DELIGHT

1 cup milk
2 tablespoons potato starch
1/8 teaspoon salt
1 tablespoon lemon juice
1 egg
2 1/2 tablespoons honey
1 mashed banana

Mix potato starch with 1/4 cup milk. Add to remainder of milk which has been scalded. Add honey and salt. Beat egg yolk and gradually add the hot mixture. Cook mixture 1 to 2 minutes. Add mashed bananas, lemon juice and beaten egg white. Chill.

CORNBREAD

3 tablespoons melted margarine
1 egg
1/2 teaspoon salt
1 cup cornmeal
1 cup buttermilk
1/2 teaspoon soda

Mix all ingredients together. Pour into greased cake pan and bake at 400 for 35 to 40 minutes.

NOODLES

1/3 cup rice flour
1/2 teaspoon baking powder
1/4 teaspoon salt
1 egg

Mix together. Knead into dough. Roll dough 1/8" thick. Dry 10 minutes and cut into strips. Dry two hours more. Store in refrigerator.

APPLE MUFFINS

2 cups rice flour
1/3 cup honey
4 teaspoon baking powder
1 teaspoon cinnamon
3/4 cup water
1/3 cup dry milk
1 egg
1 teaspoon salt
1 cup chopped apple pieces
1/4 cup vegetable oil

Mix all ingredients and pour into buttered muffin tins. On top of this sprinkle a mixture of:

1/3 cup brown sugar
1/3 cup nuts
1/2 teaspoon cinnamon
Bake at 350 until done.

RICE BISCUITS

1 cup rice flour
2 teaspoon baking powder
1/2 cup skim milk
1 teaspoon honey
1/2 teaspoon salt
2 tablespoons vegetable oil

Mix and form into biscuits. Place on greased cookie sheet. Stand 10 minutes before baking. Bake at 350 for 30 to 35 minutes.

Pumpkin Bread

1/2cup brown sugar

1 cup cooked pumpkin

1/2 cup sunflower oil

1 cup honey

2 eggs

Combine all five of these ingredients. Then combine the ingredients below:

2 cups rice flour

1 teaspoon baking soda

1 teaspoon cinnamon

1/4 teaspoon lemon peel

1/2 teaspoon each of salt, nutmeg, ginger and cloves.

Put the two mixtures together and mix well. Stir in:

1 cup raisins

1/4 cup water

1/2 cup chopped nuts

Pour into well-greased loaf pan 9 x 5 x 3. Bake at 350 for 1 1/2 hours.

Honey Peanut Butter Candy

1 cup honey
1 cup peanut butter
1 1/2 cup dry milk

Mix together. Drop by teaspoon on waxed paper. Refrigerate.

Pineapple Pudding

1 1/4 cup scalded milk
1/4 cup cold milk
2 tablespoons potato starch
2 egg whites
2 tablespoons honey
1/8 teaspoon salt
1/4 cup crushed, drained pineapple

Add potato starch to the cold milk and stir this into the hot milk. Add honey and salt and cook until thickened. Add crushed pineapple and remove from the stove. Fold in the stiffly beaten egg whites. Chill and serve. Any fruit may be substituted for the pineapple.

CRESCENTS

1 cup potato starch

1/2 cup honey

1/4 teaspoon salt

2 teaspoons baking powder

4 tablespoons shortening

5 tablespoons water

1/2 teaspoon vanilla

1/2 cup shredded coconut

Place dry ingredients in mixing bowl and work shortening into them. Add water and flavoring. Work dough to a smooth consistency that holds together without being sticky. Add coconut. Form into small crescents and place on cookie sheet. Bake at 350 for 12 to 15 minutes.

CHIFFON CAKE

1 cup rice flour

1/2 teaspoon salt

1 1/2 teaspoon baking powder

3/8 cup water

3/4 cup honey

1/4 cup salad oil

1 teaspoon vanilla

3 egg yolks

Grated rind of one lemon

Sift dry ingredients together. Add rest of ingredients and beat for one minute on electric mixer. Place 3 egg whites and 1/4 tsp. cream of tartar in separate bowl and beat until stiff. Fold egg whites into above mixture. Pour into 8 x 8 ungreased pan. Bake at 350 for 25 minutes.

PEANUT BUTTER SQUARES

1/3 cup margarine

1/4 cup peanut butter

2 1/2 cups puffed rice

1/4 cup brown sugar

1/4 cup honey

Combine all ingredients except rice in saucepan. Bring to a boil over medium heat; reduce heat, cook for 2 minutes. Mix in puffed rice. Press into 8" square pan. Chill.

Rice Cake

1 1/2 cup rice flour
2 teaspoons baking powder
1/3 cup butter
3/4 cup honey
1/4 teaspoon salt
1 teaspoon vanilla
2 eggs (separated)
2/3 cup milk

Cream butter and honey together. Add salt, egg yolk and vanilla. Beat well. Sift rice flour with baking powder. Add together. Let stand 10 minutes before folding in stiff beaten egg whites. Pour into 8 x 8 greased pan. Bake 40 to 45 minutes at 350. Top with frosting below.

Broiled Pecan Frosting

1/2 cup honey
2 tablespoons butter
1/2 cup pecans
2 tablespoons milk

Mix and spread over warm cake. Broil until hot and bubbly, (1 to 2 minutes).

RICE FLOUR PANCAKES

1 cup rice flour
1/2 teaspoon salt
2 eggs
2 tablespoons honey
2 teaspoons baking powder
3/4 cup milk
2 tablespoons oil

Mix together and cook on griddle as regular pancakes.

RICE FLOUR RAISIN MUFFINS

1 1/2 cup rice flour
2 teaspoon baking powder
1/2 tsp salt
1/2 cup raisins
1/2 cup honey
1/3 cup milk
1 egg
1/4 cup melted butter

Mix all ingredients. Spoon into buttered muffin pan 2/3 full. Bake at 350 for 15 minutes.

ZAMBOZETTI

12 ounces cooked noodles
1 chopped onion
2 cups tomato juice
1 1/21 Ib. hamburger
8 oz. cubed cheddar cheese

Brown hamburger and drain. Mix cooked noodles and hamburger together in a 13 x 9 casserole dish. Add chopped onion and cubed cheese. Stir well to mix all ingredients. Salt and pepper to taste. Pour 2 cups tomato juice over casserole to make moist. Dot with butter and let stand one hour before baking. Bake one hour at 400 degrees.

RICE FLOUR BANANA BREAD

2 1/2 cups rice flour
4 tablespoons baking powder
1 teaspoon vanilla
2 tablespoons honey
2 teaspoons baking powder
3/4 cup milk
2 tablespoons oil

Mix together and cook on griddle as regular pancakes.

1 1/2 cup mashed banana

2 beaten eggs

3/4 cup honey

1 teaspoon salt

1 cup nuts

1/2 cup milk

3 tablespoons vegetable oil

Combine all ingredients and stir until mixed. Pour into greased loaf pan 9 x 5 x 3. Bake at 350 for 1 to 1 1/2 hours. Check for doneness by inserting toothpick until it comes out clean.

Pizza

3 cups cooked rice

2 eggs

1 cup Mozzarella cheese

Mix together and press into a 12" pizza pan. Bake at 450 for 20 minutes.

2 cans tomato sauce (watch for brand with no sugar)

1/2 tsp. oregano

1/2 tsp. basil

1/2 tsp. garlic powder

1/2tsp. salt

Mix together for sauce. Pour and spread over cooked crust.

Top with:

1 cup Mozzarella cheese

2 tablespoons Parmesan cheese

    Bake until done. You may add your own favorite toppings but use caution. With ground beef, brown until fully cooked, drain fat from it and press fats and oils out of it with paper towels before putting on pizza.

CHAPTER

14

How long does it take to be healthy and normal again?

I can't answer this. Age, attitude, eating habits, daily stress, degree of health problem, exercise and rest all had much to do with the time needed to rebuild my body. I have heard from others who experienced almost immediate changes, and I've also heard from some who had gone well over a year without noticeable improvement. It seems to vary with everyone. I know that my condition was very bad, and it took me over four years to be in top health. I've seen others do the same much quicker.

Can this work for other degenerative conditions like arthritis, diabetes, muscular dystrophy, etc?

I know people with all of these conditions who have been helped by a nutritional program. I feel we need to treat all degenerative diseases as being caused by what we have done to ourselves nutritionally. You will hear many doctors say that it won't help and you will hear many nutritionists say that it will help. Since I can't prove it would help and there doesn't seem to be a straight out yes or no answer to it, I know that if I had any health problem, I would give nutrition a long, sincere effort.

What does your doctor say about what you are doing?

At first, doctors discouraged me from trying nutrition because they felt it wouldn't help. They told me I was wasting my money. They didn't mention the money I had wasted with them. I'm not doing what they were taught. There is no scientifically proven fact to it. There is no way for scientists to run double blind studies on it. But that never mattered to me.

Will this help vision?

It sure helped mine! When my health was really bad, I had to wear a patch on one eye to watch TV or read due to double vision. I had a hard time passing a vision test for driving, even with my glasses. A medical friend of mine says it's due to normal eye changes. I don't know too many people who "suffer" from improvement of vision. I choose to believe that my good vision comes from my good health habits.

Do you use physical therapy?

Yes! I work, mow the lawn, ride the bicycle, go dancing, walk, play in a band, stay active, and I quit when I'm tired. I do not use trained therapists to exercise me. How would they know what I need? How do they know how much energy I have? How can they tell when I'm tired?

Are you in remission?

Again, I don't think so. Most doctors will tell you I am in remission. I know that the doctors who knew me when I was really down are amazed at my present condition and simply say, "I don't know what you did, but keep doing it."

The treatment I have chosen is not medically documented, therefore doctors don't recommend the use of it. I do know that remissions come and go without anyone being able to control them. Yet I can control my health. If I am away from home and have to rely on restaurant foods, if I can't get the rest I need, or if I forget to take my supplements, there is a noticeable change in my condition. I can correct it myself by doing what I feel is needed. I haven't met anyone in a remission who could control their health condition. If it is a remission, it's a remission I control.

Will you call or write my friend who has MS and talk to them about this?

No! Consistently, when I contact someone, they feel I am trying to force this on them. The individual person has to want it enough to look for the answers on their own. This is the first step of having the right attitude. I really believe that attitude is at least 90% of the recovery.

How did your family deal with your health when you were really down?

My parents were supportive and willing to help me in trying anything. When I became dedicated to nutrition, they decided I was crazy! They were too much help. They didn't make me do things for myself.

My first wife nursed me for three years and divorced me. Who could blame her? I was belligerent, argumentative, angry and difficult to live with. This seems to be common to everyone with MS. It's a hard condition to live with either as the victim or family of the victim. MS victims need to be told that anger is a normal response, and then given some help in dealing with it. When you are getting worse all the time and there's nothing to do about it, you have a tendency to be irritable!

What supplements do you take?

I take what I need. It changes daily, and I can feel the changes. There is no way of putting an amount on any of the nutrients. It constantly varies. This is why I simply take large amounts and let my body use what it needs. No one can tell what is needed. Only your body knows.

I've been on a vitamin and diet therapy for eighteen months and I'm not any better. Why haven't I improved?

Maybe you have. Perhaps, if you hadn't been treating yourself nutritionally, you would be much worse. Maybe you will be like me and need three to four years. Maybe it really won't work for you. Isn't it worth trying?

When you first started using a nutritional approach, did you feel worse than before or suffer from any problems?

Yes! I think it is important to remember that my health condition was a result of a lifetime of poor nutrition. I could not expect overnight results. I also had to realize that the process of rebuilding meant letting my body discard bad cells and replace them with good cells. I had to understand I would have varying symptoms as my body did this.

Common problems when one starts using a nutritional approach are: headaches, fever, colds, skin blemishes, dizziness, bowel problems, weakness, disinclination to exercise, nervousness, irritability, mental depression and tiredness. I suffered from most of these symptoms when I first started using nutrition. I wasn't alarmed because I was expecting some effects, and I also knew they wouldn't last long. Good nutrition can't harm you. Anything that happens is for the good.

CHAPTER

15

So that's it! That's what happened to Vince Stephens. I decided that with MS there was nothing wrong with my brain, nothing wrong with my muscles, and nothing wrong with my nerves. I don't believe MS is a disease. I believe it is just something that can happen to the body when it's not fed properly. Doctors feel MS is caused by a virus. I don't agree. My body simply needed better nutrition and I needed an attitude adjustment. I don't believe a "cure" will ever be found for any of these degenerative conditions. Our hospitals are full, our nursing homes are full, and we see sick people walking down the street every day. All that most of them need is just something good to eat.

I am against electric wheelchairs, medical treatment, physical therapy, snake venom, gold injections, hair analysis, blood testing, and every other form of outside treatment for MS. I honestly believe the control of MS must come from the individual. I even accept the fact that many are content with their MS. I don't understand it, but I accept it!

I have good reason to be against all these things. When I

wonder if I'm wrong, I always remember the time I passed my former pharmacist on the street. She was amazed to see me. She wasn't amazed because I was better. She was amazed that I was alive. She said that the combination of medications I had been taking should have killed me. I asked her why she filled the prescriptions when she knew they could kill me. She said, "I'm only responsible for selling what your doctor prescribes".

Throughout this book I avoided using names or places. It was done for many reasons. I realized that some of the people involved don't want their name associated with everything I've been through.

When I first spoke of looking for new approaches to treat my MS, I talked about hearing of a woman in Kansas City who used a nutritional approach to go from bedridden to healthy. I got a call from that woman. Someone had told her about me. She had never had the health recovery as I was told. She heard of my recovery and was wanting to know what I had done to control my MS. Her condition was bad and she was wanting my help. Someone had used her name and made up the entire story about her recovery to sell supplements. I am amazed that my present good health is due in part to someone's lie. This is why I understand skepticism from all directions. I still get letters from people offering a "cure" for MS, which reminds me how confusing it can get when you're looking for answers.

I have not tried to write this as the solution or the answer for MS. I have simply tried to explain what I have done myself. I do have a strong belief of it helping anyone who will let it help, and with any degenerative condition. Please don't call me and ask if I think this will work for you. I know it worked for me. Weather it will works for you depends on you! I am enjoying life at its best. I will not go back down. I wish the same good health for you. God Bless!

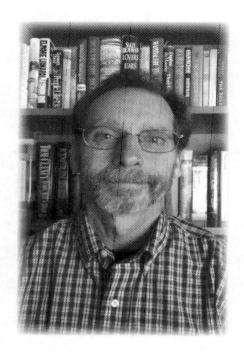

Vincent Stephens, Jr. grew up in Central Kansas. He was an Eagle Scout and one of six from the USA who attended the 1966 Boy Scout World Jamboree in Scotland. As a teenager he built and raced fast cars. He learned to play string bass in school and played in the local symphony. He also played bass guitar and recorded with a popular Midwest rock band. He owned and operated several small businesses including an auto parts store and machine shop. Today, at age 65, he still drives fast cars and performs several times a month with his current band.

Printed in the United States
By Bookmasters